Copyright © 2021

Table of Contents

16 Foods to Eat on a Ketogenic Diet

The ketogenic diet has become popular. Studies have found that this very low carb, high fat diet is effective for weight loss, diabetes, and epilepsy.

There's also early evidence to show that it may be beneficial for certain cancers, Alzheimer's disease, and other diseases, too.

Still, higher quality research on the diet is still needed to determine its long-term safety and efficacy.

A ketogenic diet typically limits carbs to 20 to 50 grams per day. While this may seem challenging, many nutritious foods can easily fit into this way of eating.

Here are some healthy foods to eat on a ketogenic diet.

1. Seafood

Fish and shellfish are very keto-friendly foods. Salmon and other fish are rich in B vitamins, potassium, and selenium, yet virtually carb-free.

However, the carbs in different types of shellfish vary. For instance, while shrimp and most crabs contain no carbs, other types of shellfish do.

While these shellfish can still be included on a ketogenic diet, it's important to account for these carbs when you're trying to stay within a narrow range.

Here are the carb counts for 3.5-ounce (100-gram) servings of some popular types of shellfish:

- clams: 4 grams

- mussels: 4 grams

- octopus: 4 grams

- oysters: 3 grams

- squid: 3 grams

Salmon, sardines, mackerel, and other fatty fish are very high in omega-3 fats, which have been found to lower insulin levels and increase insulin sensitivity in people who have overweight and obesity.

In addition, frequent fish intake has been linked to a decreased risk of disease and improved cognitive health.

The American Heart Association recommends consuming 1 to 2 seafood meals every week.

SUMMARY

Many types of seafood are carb-free or very low in carbs. Fish and shellfish are also good sources of vitamins, minerals, and omega-3s.

2. Low-carb vegetables

Non-starchy vegetables are low in calories and carbs, but high in many nutrients, including vitamin C and several minerals.

Vegetables and other plants contain fiber, which your body doesn't digest and absorb like other carbs.

Therefore, look at their digestible (or net) carb count, which is total carbs minus fiber. The term "net carbs" simply refers to carbs that are absorbed by the body.

Note that net carbs and their effects on the body are somewhat controversial, and more research is needed.

Many vegetables contain very few net carbs. However, consuming one serving of "starchy" vegetables like potatoes, yams, or beets could put you over your entire carb limit for the day.

The net carb count for non-starchy vegetables ranges from less than 1 gram for 1 cup of raw spinach to 7 grams for 1 cup of cooked Brussels sprouts.

Vegetables also contain antioxidants that help protect against free radicals, which are unstable molecules that can cause cell damage.

What's more, cruciferous vegetables like kale, broccoli, and cauliflower have been linked to decreased cancer and heart disease risk.

Low carb veggies make great substitutes for higher carb foods.

For instance:

- cauliflower can be used to mimic rice or mashed potatoes

- "zoodles" can be created from zucchini

- spaghetti squash is a natural substitute for spaghetti

Here are some examples of keto-friendly vegetables to include in your eating plan.

Keto vegetable list:

- asparagus

- avocado

- broccoli

- cabbage

- cauliflower

- cucumber

- green beans

- eggplant

- kale

- lettuce

- olives

- peppers (especially green)

- spinach

- tomatoes

- zucchini

SUMMARY

The net carbs in non-starchy vegetables range from 1 to 8 grams per cup. Vegetables are nutritious, versatile, and may help reduce the risk of disease.

3. Cheese

There are hundreds of types of cheese.

Fortunately, most are very low in carbs

and high in fat, which makes them a great fit for a ketogenic diet.

One ounce (28 grams) of cheddar cheese provides 1 gram of carbs, 6.5 grams of protein, and a good amount of calcium.

Cheese is high in saturated fat, but it hasn't been shown to increase the risk of heart disease. In fact, some studies suggest that cheese may help protect against heart disease.

Cheese also contains conjugated linoleic acid, which is a fat that has been linked to fat loss and improvements in body composition.

In addition, eating cheese regularly may help reduce the loss of muscle mass and strength that occurs with aging.

A 12-week study in older adults found that those who consumed 7 ounces (210 grams) of ricotta cheese per day experienced less muscle mass and muscle strength loss over the course of the study than others.

Here are some cheeses that are lower in carbs for a keto diet.

Keto cheese list:

- blue cheese

- brie

- camembert

- cheddar

- chevre

- colby jack

- cottage cheese

- cream cheese

- feta

- goat cheese

- halloumi

- Havarti

- Limburger

- manchego

- mascarpone

- mozzarella

- muenster

- parmesan

- pepper jack

- provalone

- romano

- string cheese

- Swiss

SUMMARY

Cheese is rich in protein, calcium, and beneficial fatty acids, yet contains a minimal amount of carbs.

4. Avocados

Avocados are incredibly healthy; 3.5 ounces (100 grams), or about one-half of a medium avocado, contain 9 grams of carbs.

However, 7 of these are fiber, so its net carb count is only 2 grams.

Avocados are high in several vitamins and minerals, including potassium, an important mineral many people may not get enough of. What's more, a higher potassium intake may help make the transition to a ketogenic diet easier.

In addition, avocados may help improve cholesterol and triglyceride levels.

One study found that participants eating one avocado per day had beneficial effects for their cardiometabolic risk factors including lower levels of LDL (bad) cholesterol.

SUMMARY

Avocados contain 2 grams of net carbs per serving and are high in fiber and several nutrients, including potassium. In addition, they may help improve heart health markers.

5. Meat and poultry

Meat and poultry are considered staple foods on a ketogenic diet.

Fresh meat and poultry contain no carbs and are rich in B vitamins and several important minerals.

They're also a great source of high-quality protein, which has been shown to help preserve muscle mass during a very low carb diet.

One study in older women found that consuming a diet high in fatty meat led to HDL (good) cholesterol levels that were 5% higher than on a low fat, high carb diet.

It's best to choose grass-fed meat, if possible. That's because animals that eat grass produce meat with higher amounts of omega-3 fats, conjugated linoleic acid, and antioxidants than meat from grain-fed animals.

SUMMARY

Meat and poultry do not contain carbs and are rich in high-quality protein and several nutrients. Grass-fed meat is the healthiest choice.

6. Eggs

Eggs are one of the healthiest and most versatile foods on the planet.

One large egg contains less than 1 gram of carbs and about 6 grams of protein, making eggs an ideal food for a ketogenic lifestyle.

In addition, eggs have been shown to trigger hormones that increase feelings of fullness and satiety.

It's important to eat the entire egg, as most of an egg's nutrients are found in the yolk. This includes the antioxidants lutein and zeaxanthin, which help protect eye health.

Although egg yolks are high in cholesterol, consuming them doesn't raise blood cholesterol levels in most people. In fact, eggs appear to modify the size of LDL particles in a way that reduces the risk of heart disease.

SUMMARY

Eggs contain less than 1 gram of carbs each and can help keep you full for hours. They're also high in several nutrients and may help protect eye and heart health.

7. Coconut oil

Coconut oil has unique properties that make it well suited for a ketogenic diet.

To begin with, it contains medium-chain triglycerides (MCTs). Unlike long-chain fats, MCTs are taken up directly by the liver and converted into ketones or used as a rapid source of energy.

In fact, coconut oil has been used to increase ketone levels in people with Alzheimer's disease and other disorders of the brain and nervous system.

The main fatty acid in coconut oil is lauric acid, a slightly longer-chain fat. It has been suggested that coconut oil's mix of MCTs and lauric acid may promote a sustained level of ketosis.

What's more, coconut oil may help adults with obesity lose weight and belly fat.

In one study, men who ate 2 tablespoons (30 mL) of coconut oil per day lost 1 inch (2.5 cm), on average, from their waistlines without making any other dietary changes.

SUMMARY

Coconut oil is rich in MCTs, which can increase ketone production. In addition, it may increase metabolic rate and promote the loss of weight and belly fat.

8. Plain Greek yogurt and cottage cheese

Plain Greek yogurt and cottage cheese are healthy, high protein foods.

While they contain some carbs, they can still be included in a ketogenic lifestyle in moderation.

A half cup (105 grams) of plain Greek yogurt provides 4 grams of carbs and 9 grams of protein. That amount of cottage cheese provides 5 grams of carbs and 11 grams of protein.

Both yogurt and cottage cheese have been shown to help decrease appetite and promote feelings of fullness.

Either one makes a tasty snack on its own. However, both can also be combined with chopped nuts, cinnamon, or other spices for a quick and easy keto treat.

SUMMARY

Both plain Greek yogurt and cottage cheese contain 5 grams of carbs per serving. Studies have shown that they help reduce appetite and promote fullness.

9. Olive oil

Olive oil provides impressive benefits for your heart.

It's high in oleic acid, a monounsaturated fat that has been found to decrease heart disease risk factors in many studies.

In addition, extra-virgin olive oil is high in antioxidants known as phenols. These compounds further protect heart health by decreasing inflammation and improving artery function.

As a pure fat source, olive oil contains no carbs. It's an ideal base for salad dressings and healthy mayonnaise.

Because it isn't as stable as saturated fats at high temperatures, it's best to use olive oil for low-heat cooking or add it to foods after they've been cooked.

SUMMARY

Extra-virgin olive oil is high in heart-healthy monounsaturated fats and antioxidants. It's ideal for salad dressings, mayonnaise, and adding to cooked foods.

10. Nuts and seeds

Nuts and seeds are healthy, high fat, and low-carb foods.

Frequent nut consumption has been linked to a reduced risk of heart disease, certain cancers, depression, and other chronic diseases.

Furthermore, nuts and seeds are high in fiber, which can help you feel full and absorb fewer calories overall.

Although all nuts and seeds are low in net carbs, the amount varies quite a bit among the different types.

Here are the carb counts for 1 ounce (28 grams) of some popular nuts and seeds:

- almonds: 2 grams net carbs (6 grams total carbs)

- Brazil nuts: 1 gram net carbs (3 grams total carbs)

- cashews: 8 grams net carbs (9 grams total carbs)

- macadamia nuts: 2 grams net carbs (4 grams total carbs)

- pecans: 2 grams net carbs (4 grams total carbs)

- pistachios: 5 grams net carbs (8 grams total carbs)

- walnuts: 2 grams net carbs (4 grams total carbs)

- chia seeds: 1 gram net carbs (12 grams total carbs)

- flaxseeds: 0 grams net carbs (8 grams total carbs)

- pumpkin seeds: 3 grams net carbs (5 grams total carbs)

- sesame seeds: 3 grams net carbs (7 grams total carbs)

SUMMARY

Nuts and seeds are heart-healthy, high in fiber, and may lead to healthier aging. They provide 0 to 8 grams of net carbs per ounce.

11. Berries

Most fruits are too high in carbs to include on a ketogenic diet, but berries are an exception.

Berries are low in carbs and high in fiber. In fact, raspberries and blackberries contain as much fiber as digestible carbs.

These tiny fruits are loaded with antioxidants that have been credited with reducing inflammation and protecting against disease.

Here are the carb counts for 3.5 ounces (100 grams) of some berries:

• blackberries: 11 grams net carbs (16 grams total carbs)

• blueberries: 9 grams net carbs (12 grams total carbs)

• raspberries: 6 grams net carbs (12 grams total carbs)

• strawberries: 7 grams net carbs (9 grams total carbs)

SUMMARY

Berries are rich in nutrients that may reduce the risk of disease. They provide 5 to 12 grams of net carbs per 3.5-ounce serving.

12. Butter and cream

Butter and cream are good fats to include on a ketogenic diet. Each contains only trace amounts of carbs per serving.

For many years, butter and cream were believed to cause or contribute to heart disease due to their high saturated fat contents. However, several large studies have shown that, for most people, saturated fat isn't linked to heart disease.

In fact, some studies suggest that a moderate consumption of high fat dairy may possibly reduce the risk of heart attack and stroke.

Like other fatty dairy products, butter and cream are rich in conjugated linoleic acid, the fatty acid that may promote fat loss.

SUMMARY

Butter and cream are nearly carb-free and appear to have neutral or beneficial effects on heart health when consumed in moderation.

13. Shirataki noodles

Shirataki noodles are a fantastic addition to a ketogenic diet. You can find them near the produce at grocery stores or online.

They contain less than 1 gram of net carbs and 15 calories per serving because they're mainly water.

In fact, these noodles are made from a viscous fiber called glucomannan, which can absorb up to 50 times its weight in water.

Viscous fiber forms a gel that slows down food's movement through your digestive tract. This can help decrease hunger and blood sugar spikes, making it beneficial for weight loss and diabetes management.

Shirataki noodles come in a variety of shapes, including rice, fettuccine, and linguine. They can be substituted for regular noodles in all types of recipes.

SUMMARY

Shirataki noodles contain less than 1 gram of carbs per serving. Their viscous fiber helps slow down the movement of food through your digestive tract, which promotes fullness and stable blood sugar levels.

14. Olives

Olives provide the same health benefits as olive oil, only in solid form.

Oleuropein, the main antioxidant found in olives, has anti-inflammatory properties and may protect your cells from damage.

In addition, in vitro studies suggest that consuming olives may help prevent bone loss and decrease blood pressure, though no human trials are available yet.

Olives vary in carb content due to their size. However, half of their carbs come from fiber, so their digestible carb content is very low.

Ten olives (34 grams) contain 2 grams of total carbs and 1 gram of fiber. This works out to a net carb count of about 1 gram depending on the size.

SUMMARY

Olives are rich in antioxidants that may help protect heart and bone health.

They contain 1 gram of net carbs per ounce.

15. Unsweetened coffee and tea

Coffee and tea are healthy, carb-free drinks.

They contain caffeine, which increases your metabolism and may help improve your physical performance, alertness, and mood.

What's more, coffee and tea drinkers have been shown to have a significantly reduced risk of diabetes. In fact, those with the highest coffee intake have the lowest risk for developing diabetes.

Adding heavy cream to coffee or tea is fine but stay away from "light" coffee and tea lattes. These are typically made with nonfat milk and contain high carb flavorings.

SUMMARY

Unsweetened coffee and tea contain no carbs and can help boost your metabolic rate, as well as physical and mental performance. They can also reduce your risk for diabetes.

16. Dark chocolate and cocoa powder

Dark chocolate and cocoa are delicious sources of antioxidants.

In fact, cocoa provides at least as much antioxidant activity as any other fruit, including blueberries and acai berries.

Dark chocolate contains flavanols, which may help reduce the risk of heart disease by lowering blood pressure and keeping arteries healthy.

Somewhat surprisingly, chocolate can be part of a ketogenic diet. However, it's important to choose dark chocolate that contains a minimum of 70% cocoa solids, preferably more, and eat in moderation.

One ounce (28 grams) of unsweetened chocolate (100% cocoa) has 3 grams of net carbs.

SUMMARY

Dark chocolate and cocoa powder are high in antioxidants and may help reduce the risk of heart disease.

The bottom line

A ketogenic diet can be used to achieve weight loss, blood sugar management, and other health-related goals.

Fortunately, it can include a wide variety of nutritious, tasty, and versatile foods that allow you to remain within your daily carb range.

To reap all the health benefits of a ketogenic diet, consume keto-friendly foods on a regular basis.

Food Fix: Keto Basics

15 Health Conditions That May Benefit From a Ketogenic Diet

Ketogenic diets have become incredibly popular.

Early research suggests this high-fat, very low-carb diet may benefit several health conditions.

Although some of the evidence is from case studies and animal research, results from human controlled studies are also promising.

Here are 15 health conditions that may benefit from a ketogenic diet.

1. Epilepsy

Epilepsy is a disease that causes seizures due to excessive brain activity.

Anti-seizure medications are effective for some people with epilepsy. However, others don't respond to the drugs or can't tolerate their side effects.

Of all the conditions that may benefit from a ketogenic diet, epilepsy has by far the most evidence supporting it. In fact, there are several dozen studies on the topic.

Research shows that seizures typically improve in about 50% of epilepsy patients who follow the classic ketogenic diet. This is also known as a 4:1 ketogenic diet because it provides 4 times as much fat as protein and carbs combined.

The modified Atkins diet (MAD) is based on a considerably less restrictive 1:1 ratio of fat to protein and carbs. It has been shown to be equally effective for seizure control in most adults and children older than two years of age.

The ketogenic diet may also have benefits on the brain beyond seizure control.

For example, when researchers examined the brain activity of children with epilepsy, they found improvements in various brain patterns in 65% of those following a ketogenic diet — regardless of whether they had fewer seizures.

BOTTOM LINE:

Ketogenic diets have been shown to reduce seizure frequency and severity in many children and adults with epilepsy who don't respond well to drug therapy.

2. Metabolic Syndrome

Metabolic syndrome, sometimes referred to as prediabetes, is characterized by insulin resistance.

You can be diagnosed with metabolic syndrome if you meet any 3 of these criteria:

- Large waistline: 35 inches (89 cm) or higher in women and 40 inches (102 cm) or higher in men.

- Elevated triglycerides: 150 mg/dl (1.7 mmol/L) or higher.

- Low HDL cholesterol: Less than 40 mg/dL (1.04 mmol/L) in men and less than 50 mg/dL (1.3 mmol/L) in women.

- High blood pressure: 130/85 mm Hg or higher.

- Elevated fasting blood sugar: 100 mg/dL (5.6 mmol/L) or higher.

People with metabolic syndrome are at increased risk of diabetes, heart disease and other serious disorders related to insulin resistance.

Fortunately, following a ketogenic diet may improve many features of metabolic syndrome. Improvements may include better cholesterol values, as well as reduced blood sugar and blood pressure.

In a controlled 12-week study, people with metabolic syndrome on a calorie-restricted ketogenic diet lost 14% of their body fat. They decreased triglycerides by more than 50% and experienced several other improvements in health markers.

BOTTOM LINE:

Ketogenic diets may reduce abdominal obesity, triglycerides, blood pressure and blood sugar in people with metabolic syndrome.

3. Glycogen Storage Disease

People with glycogen storage disease (GSD) lack one of the enzymes involved in storing glucose (blood sugar) as glycogen or breaking glycogen down into glucose. There are several types of GSD, each based on the enzyme that is missing.

Typically, this disease is diagnosed in childhood. Symptoms vary depending on the type of GSD, and may include poor growth, fatigue, low blood sugar, muscle cramps and an enlarged liver.

GSD patients are often advised to consume high-carb foods at frequent intervals so glucose is always available to the body.

However, early research suggests that a ketogenic diet may benefit people with some forms of GSD.

For example, GSD III, also known as Forbes-Cori disease, affects the liver and muscles. Ketogenic diets may help relieve symptoms by providing ketones that can be used as an alternate fuel source.

GSD V, also known as McArdle disease, affects the muscles and is characterized by a limited ability to exercise.

In one case, a man with GSD V followed a ketogenic diet for one year. Depending on the level of exertion required, he experienced a dramatic 3-

to 10-fold increase in exercise tolerance.

However, controlled studies are needed to confirm the potential benefits of ketogenic diet therapy in people with glycogen storage disease.

BOTTOM LINE:

People with certain types of glycogen storage disease may experience a dramatic improvement in symptoms while following a ketogenic diet. However, more research is needed.

4. Polycystic Ovary Syndrome (PCOS)

Polycystic ovary syndrome (PCOS) is a disease marked by hormonal dysfunction that often results in irregular periods and infertility.

One of its hallmarks is insulin resistance, and many women with PCOS are obese and have a hard time losing weight. Women with PCOS are also at an increased risk for type 2 diabetes.

Those who meet the criteria for metabolic syndrome tend to have symptoms that affect their appearance. Effects may include increased facial hair, acne and other signs of masculinity related to higher testosterone levels.

A lot of anecdotal evidence can be found online. However, only a few published studies confirm the benefits of low-carb and ketogenic diets for PCOS.

In a 6-month study of eleven women with PCOS following a ketogenic diet, weight loss averaged 12%. Fasting insulin also declined by 54% and reproductive hormone levels improved. Two women suffering from infertility became pregnant.

BOTTOM LINE:

Women with PCOS following a ketogenic diet may experience weight loss, reduction in insulin levels and improvement in reproductive hormone function.

5. Diabetes

People with diabetes often experience impressive reductions in blood sugar levels on a ketogenic diet. This is true of both type 1 and type 2 diabetes.

Indeed, dozens of controlled studies show that a very low-carb diet helps control blood sugar and may also provide other health benefits.

In a 16-week study, 17 of 21 people on a ketogenic diet were able to discontinue or decrease diabetes medication dosage. Study participants also lost an average of 19 pounds (8.7 kg) and reduced their waist size, triglycerides and blood pressure.

In a 3-month study comparing a ketogenic diet to a moderate-carb diet, people in the ketogenic group averaged a 0.6% decrease in HbA1c.

12% of participants achieved an HbA1c below 5.7%, which is considered normal.

BOTTOM LINE:

Ketogenic diets have been shown to reduce blood sugar in people with diabetes. In some cases, values return to a normal range, and medications can be discontinued or reduced.

6. Some Cancers

Cancer is one of the leading causes of death worldwide.

In recent years, scientific research has suggested that a ketogenic diet may help some types of cancer when used along with traditional treatments such as chemotherapy, radiation and surgery.

Many researchers note that elevated blood sugar, obesity and type 2 diabetes are linked to breast and other cancers. They suggest that restricting carbs in order to lower blood sugar and insulin levels may help prevent tumor growth.

Mice studies show ketogenic diets may reduce the progression of several types of cancer, including cancers that have spread to other parts of the body.

However, some experts believe the ketogenic diet may be particularly beneficial for brain cancer.

Case studies and patient data analyses have found improvements in various types of brain cancer, including glioblastoma multiforme (GBM) — the most common and aggressive form of brain cancer.

One study found 6 out of 7 GBM patients had a modest response to an unrestricted-calorie ketogenic diet combined with an anti-cancer drug. Researchers noted that the diet is safe but probably of limited use alone.

Some researchers report preservation of muscle mass and slowed tumor growth in cancer patients who follow a ketogenic diet in conjunction with radiation or other anti-cancer therapies.

Although it may not have a significant impact on disease progression in advanced and terminal cancers, the ketogenic diet has been shown to be safe in these patients and potentially improve quality of life.

Randomized clinical studies need to examine how ketogenic diets affect cancer patients. Several are currently underway or in the recruiting process.

BOTTOM LINE:

Animal and human research suggests ketogenic diets may benefit people with certain cancers, when combined with other therapies.

7. Autism

Autism spectrum disorder (ASD) refers to a condition characterized by problems with communication, social interaction and, in some cases, repetitive behaviors. Usually diagnosed in childhood, it is treated with speech therapy and other therapies.

Early research in young mice and rats suggests ketogenic diets may be helpful for improving ASD behavior patterns.

Autism shares some features with epilepsy, and many people with autism experience seizures related to the over-excitement of brain cells.

Studies show that ketogenic diets reduce brain cell over-stimulation in mouse models of autism. What's more, they appear to benefit behavior regardless of changes in seizure activity.

A pilot study of 30 children with autism found that 18 showed some improvement in symptoms after following a cyclical ketogenic diet for 6 months.

In one case study, a young girl with autism who followed a gluten-free, dairy-free ketogenic diet for several years experienced dramatic improvements. These included resolution of morbid obesity and a 70-point increase in IQ.

Randomized controlled studies exploring the effects of a ketogenic diet in ASD patients are now underway or in the recruiting process.

BOTTOM LINE:

Early research suggests some people with autism spectrum disorders may experience improvements in behavior when ketogenic diets are used in combination with other therapies.

8. Parkinson's Disease

Parkinson's Disease (PD) is a nervous system disorder characterized by low levels of the signaling molecule dopamine.

The lack of dopamine causes several symptoms, including tremor, impaired posture, stiffness and difficulty walking and writing.

Because of the ketogenic diet's protective effects on the brain and nervous system, it's being explored as a potential complementary therapy for PD.

Feeding ketogenic diets to rats and mice with PD led to increased energy production, protection against nerve damage and improved motor function.

In an uncontrolled study, seven people with PD followed a classic 4:1 ketogenic diet. After 4 weeks, five of them averaged a 43% improvement in symptoms.

The effects of a ketogenic diet on PD is another area that needs controlled studies.

BOTTOM LINE:

The ketogenic diet has shown promise in improving symptoms of Parkinson's disease in both animal and human studies. However, high-quality research is needed.

9. Obesity

Many studies show that very low-carb, ketogenic diets are often more effective for weight loss than calorie-restricted or low-fat diets.

What's more, they typically provide other health improvements as well.

In a 24-week study, men who followed a ketogenic diet lost twice as much fat as men who ate a low-fat diet.

In addition, the ketogenic group's triglycerides dropped significantly, and their HDL ("good") cholesterol increased. The low-fat group had a smaller drop in triglycerides and a decrease in HDL cholesterol.

Ketogenic diets' ability to reduce hunger is one of the reasons why they work so well for weight loss.

A large analysis found that very low-carb, calorie-restricted ketogenic diets help people feel less hungry than standard calorie-restricted diets..

Even when people on a ketogenic diet are allowed to eat all they want, they generally end up eating fewer calories due to the appetite-suppressing effects of ketosis.

In a study of obese men who consumed either a calorie-unrestricted ketogenic or moderate-carb diet, those in the ketogenic group had significantly less hunger, took in fewer calories and lost 31% more weight than the moderate-carb group.

BOTTOM LINE:

Studies have found that ketogenic diets are very effective for weight loss in obese people. This is largely due to their powerful appetite-suppressing effects.

10. GLUT1 Deficiency Syndrome

Glucose transporter 1 (GLUT1) deficiency syndrome, a rare genetic disorder, involves deficiency of a special protein that helps move blood sugar into the brain.

Symptoms usually begin shortly after birth and include developmental delay, difficulty with movement and sometimes seizures.

Unlike glucose, ketones don't require this protein to cross from the blood to the brain. Therefore, the ketogenic diet can provide an alternative fuel source that these children's brains can use effectively.

Indeed, ketogenic diet therapy seems to improve several symptoms of the disorder. Researchers report decreased seizure frequency and improvement in muscle coordination, alertness and concentration in children on ketogenic diets.

As with epilepsy, the modified Atkins diet (MAD) has been shown to provide the same benefits as the classic ketogenic diet. However, the MAD offers greater flexibility, which may result in better compliance and fewer side effects.

In a study of 10 children with GLUT1 deficiency syndrome, those who followed the MAD experienced improvements in seizures. At six months, 3 out of 6 became seizure-free.

BOTTOM LINE:

Both the classic ketogenic diet and more flexible MAD have been shown to improve seizures and other symptoms in children with GLUT1 deficiency syndrome.

11. Traumatic Brain Injury

Traumatic brain injury (TBI) most commonly results from a blow to the head, a car accident or a fall in which the head strikes the ground.

It can have devastating effects on physical function, memory and personality. Unlike cells in most other organs, injured brain cells often recover very little, if at all.

Because the body's ability to use sugar following head trauma is impaired, some researchers believe the ketogenic diet may benefit people with TBI.

Rat studies suggest that starting a ketogenic diet immediately after brain injury can help reduce brain swelling, increase motor function and improve recovery. However, these effects appear to occur mainly in younger rather than older rats.

That said, controlled studies in humans are needed before any conclusions can be reached.

BOTTOM LINE:

Animal studies show that a ketogenic diet improves outcomes in rats fed a ketogenic diet after traumatic brain injury. However, there are currently no quality human studies on this.

12. Multiple Sclerosis

Multiple sclerosis (MS) damages the protective covering of nerves, which leads to communication problems between the brain and body. Symptoms include numbness and problems with balance, movement, vision and memory.

One study of MS in a mouse model found that a ketogenic diet suppressed inflammatory markers. The reduced inflammation led to improvements in memory, learning and physical function.

As with other nervous system disorders, MS appears to reduce the cells' ability to use sugar as a fuel source. A 2015 review discussed ketogenic diets' potential to assist with energy production and cell repair in MS patients.

Additionally, a recent controlled study of 48 people with MS found significant improvements in quality of life scores, cholesterol and triglycerides in the groups who followed a ketogenic diet or fasted for several days.

More studies are currently underway.

BOTTOM LINE:

Studies about the potential benefits of a ketogenic diet for treating MS are promising. However, more human studies are needed.

13. Nonalcoholic Fatty Liver Disease

Nonalcoholic fatty liver disease (NAFLD) is the most common liver disease in the Western world.

It is strongly linked to type 2 diabetes, metabolic syndrome and obesity, and there's evidence that NAFLD also improves on a very low-carb, ketogenic diet.

In a small study, 14 obese men with metabolic syndrome and NAFLD who followed a ketogenic diet for 12 weeks had significant decreases in weight, blood pressure and liver enzymes.

What's more, an impressive 93% of the men had a reduction in liver fat, and 21% achieved complete resolution of NAFLD.

BOTTOM LINE:

Ketogenic diets may be very effective at reducing liver fat and other health markers in people with nonalcoholic fatty liver disease.

14. Alzheimer's Disease

Alzheimer's disease is a progressive form of dementia characterized by plaques and tangles in the brain that impair memory.

Interestingly, Alzheimer's disease appears to share features of both epilepsy and type 2 diabetes: seizures, the inability of the brain to properly use glucose and inflammation linked to insulin resistance.

Animal studies show that a ketogenic diet improves balance and coordination but doesn't affect the amyloid plaque that is a hallmark of the disease. However, supplementing with ketone esters appears to reduce amyloid plaque.

In addition, supplementing people's diets with ketone esters or MCT oil to increase ketone levels has been shown to improve several Alzheimer's disease symptoms.

For example, one controlled study followed 152 people with Alzheimer's disease who took an MCT compound. After 45 and 90 days, this group showed improvements in mental function, while the placebo group's function declined.

Controlled studies testing the modified Atkins diet and MCT oil in people with Alzheimer's disease are currently in progress or in the recruiting stage.

BOTTOM LINE:

Several symptoms of Alzheimer's disease have been shown to improve with ketogenic diets in animal research. Human studies suggest supplementing with MCT oil or ketone esters may be beneficial.

15. Migraine Headaches

Migraine headaches typically involve severe pain, sensitivity to light and nausea.

Some studies suggest migraine headache symptoms often improve in people who follow ketogenic diets.

One observational study reported a reduction in migraine frequency and pain medication use in people following a ketogenic diet for one month.

An interesting case study of two sisters following a cyclical ketogenic diet for weight loss reported that their migraine headaches disappeared during the 4-week ketogenic cycles but returned during the 8-week transition diet cycles.

However, high-quality studies are needed to confirm the results of these reports.

BOTTOM LINE:

Some studies suggest that migraine headache frequency and severity may improve in people following a ketogenic diet.

Take Home Message

Ketogenic diets are being considered for use in several disorders due to their beneficial effects on metabolic health and the nervous system.

However, many of these impressive results come from case studies and need validation through higher-quality research, including randomized controlled trials.

With respect to cancer and several other serious diseases on this list, a ketogenic diet should be undertaken only in addition to standard therapies under the supervision of a doctor or qualified healthcare provider.

Also, no one should consider the ketogenic diet a cure for any disease or disorder on its own.

Nonetheless, the ketogenic diets' potential to improve health is very promising.